Excerpts
from a
Family
Medical
Dictionary

Excerpts from a Family Medical Dictionary

•

Rebecca Brown

THE UNIVERSITY OF WISCONSIN PRESS

The University of Wisconsin Press
1930 Monroe Street
Madison, Wisconsin 53711

www.wisc.edu/wisconsinpress/

3 Henrietta Street
London WC2E 8LU, England

5   4   3   2   1

Printed in the United States of America

Book design based on the 2001 Grey Spider Press edition, designed by
C. Christopher Stern and Jules Remedios Faye.

Library of Congress Cataloging-in-Publication Data
Brown, Rebecca, 1956–
Excerpts from a family medical dictionary / Rebecca Brown.
   p. cm.
   ISBN 0-299-18970-8 (cloth)
   1. Brown, Barbara Ann Wildman, 1928–1997—Health. 2. Cancer—Patients—
New Mexico—Biography. I. Title.
RC265.6.B76 B76   2003
362.1'96994'0092—dc21   2003005653

Terrace Books, a division of the University of Wisconsin Press, takes its name from
the Memorial Union Terrace, located at the University of Wisconsin–Madison.
Since its inception in 1907, the Wisconsin Union has provided a venue for students,
faculty, staff, and alumni to debate art, music, politics, and the issues of the day. It
is a place where theater, music, drama, dance, outdoor activities, and major
speakers are made available to the campus and the community. To learn more
about the Union, visit www.union.wisc.edu.

THE AUTHOR WISHES to thank the staff of the Gila Regional Medical Center in Silver City, New Mexico, especially the oncology and hospice folks. Every dying person and every dying person's family should always have such thoughtful, loving care.

in memory of
BARBARA ANN WILDMAN BROWN
1928–1997

CONTENTS

Excerpts
from a
Family
Medical
Dictionary

anemia

1. a condition in which there is a reduction
of red blood corpuscles or of hemoglobin,
or both, in the bloodstream. 2. lack of vigor,
lifelessness. Anemia may be only the first sign
of some other complaint; therefore the sooner
anemia is correctly diagnosed the sooner the
patient can receive the correct treatment for
whatever is causing the particular illness.

My mother started planning her trip

in January. She was going to drive her new car from Silver City, the town she'd retired to two summers before, to my sister's in L.A. She'd do this on my sister's spring break and the two of them and my sister's son would drive together up the coast to see me and Chris. But that was the year of all that rain and some of the highways collapsed so my mother called in March and said they were going to postpone the trip.

My mother had always been very big on car trips. She loved to drive. Every summer when we were growing up, she'd take us somewhere. When we lived in Spain in the 1960s—my father was in the military—she planned our family trips through France and England and Germany. When we moved back to the states, to Texas in 1966, she'd drive up north a couple times a year to visit her family in Oklahoma. She'd driven halfway across the continent more than once.

When my mother told me about postponing the trip, she also

said it would be better to do it later because by then she'd be feeling better. My mother rarely complained about feeling bad and she certainly hadn't said anything recently. When I asked her what she meant, she answered breezily that she'd caught the flu or something in the winter and hadn't quite shaken it yet. She just felt tired. I asked if she'd been to the doctor and she said yes. Her doctor had told her she needed rest.

By the time the weather had cleared and the roads had opened up, my sister was teaching again. I called my mom and suggested she fly up to see us but she didn't want to. When I pressed her she admitted she still wasn't feeling good.

I said I'd come down to see her but she put me off because, she said, she didn't want to have anyone around until she was better. I tried to take her at her word but I was worried. She said she'd go see the doctor again. This time they ran some tests but her doctor was leaving the practice and wasn't good about getting back to anyone. My mother still hadn't heard from her doctor by the time I got on a plane to go down to see her.

I flew to Albuquerque then caught a commuter flight. The commuter plane was so small it had propellers. There were eight seats and you weren't assigned one, you just took one. I'd never flown this way before and I remember looking out the window, down at the stark brown beautiful landscape. I remember seeing so clearly gray old shacks and beige dirt roads and piñon trees and bushes. I recognized the land from all the car trips Mom and I had taken but it looked different from this distance up. It didn't quite look real.

The plane seemed to gain altitude very slowly. I kept

6

wondering when we were going to get high enough that I wouldn't be able to see the details. Only when I was almost there, when the plane started its descent, did I realize it was never going to get any higher.

The Silver City airport had one runway and looked more like an outdoor basketball court than a place to land a plane. The parking lot was just wherever the cars decided to stop in the dirt.

A guy pushed some steps out to the plane and we climbed out. There were about five of us, including the pilot. We walked across the asphalt to a chain-link fence. The people gathered there to meet us started to wave. I waved to my mother. She smiled but didn't wave back. She was gripping the fence like it was holding her up.

I loaded the bags into the car and my mother handed me the keys. "Do you wanna drive while you're here?" she asked. "Sure," I said as if it was nothing: my mother had always driven.

I adjusted the mirrors in the car. When she couldn't see me looking at her, then suddenly I could see her. Her skin was pale and shiny with sweat.

"Are you OK, Mom?" I asked. "Oh, I'm fine," she said loudly. I don't know which of us she was trying to convince.

When we got to her house there was hardly any food. She'd always been one to stock up when someone was coming to see her. "Sorry there isn't much to eat," she said, "but I figured you'd know better what you want." I asked her what she'd been eating and she said she felt too tired to cook.

I found some stuff to fix us a meal and said to her, exactly the way she had to me when I was a skinny kid, "Eat! Eat! You don't eat enough to keep a bird alive!" We laughed that I was paying her back for all those years. I think we both wished that's what I was doing.

TWO MORNINGS LATER she had an appointment at the hospital with a new doctor, a cardiologist. My mother gave the directions but I drove. She had a special route that avoided the main street with the traffic and stoplights. She pointed out places where her friends lived, the library, the Garden Club and Women's Club buildings, the health food store. Some of her old liveliness came back as she was giving me the tour, but it was strange to have her telling me this from the passenger seat. We passed a restaurant she hadn't been to in a while and she said, "Oh, let's go there for lunch one day when you're here!" She sounded eager, as if this would be easy. I said I'd love to.

The cardiologist came to see patients in Silver City once a month. He examined my mother and looked at her chart then said she needed to come to the hospital in Las Cruces for more tests. Before he left, he reminded her to get her blood work done again.

Her appointment had been at 8 A.M., the first one of the day. She wanted to do some errands on the way home. I told her I could do them later, but she said she wanted to do them now. She liked doing her own errands. She was always independent. So she told me what she needed at the post office and the store and I drove to these places and dashed in while she waited in the car. When we got home we had something to eat—I made her eat—and then she took a nap.

She was still asleep when the phone rang. It was the GP who had just been assigned to her. Her former doctor had suddenly left. I told him I was her daughter who was visiting and he told me he had just seen her blood results. "Your mother is profoundly anemic," this new doctor said. Then he repeated, "*profoundly.*" He had a nice western drawl but I could hear his concern. I wished he'd been her doctor from the first. Though we'd never met, I didn't like the old one. "When can you bring her in to get her some blood?" the new one asked.

My mother had woken up when she'd heard the phone. I told her what was going on and we packed her an overnight bag and went back to the hospital. They put her in a room and hooked her up to an IV and gave her several pints of blood. After a while I could see her color coming back. She started looking ruddy again. That was good to see.

It was also good to know what had been making her so tired. After she got some blood in her she even started feeling better. "I feel so much better," she kept saying, "I can't believe how much better I feel!"

Mom hadn't met the new doctor, but when she heard who it was she was really pleased. She said some of her friends were patients of his and just adored him. She was so glad he was her doctor now. It was like, now that she knew it was just anemia and now that she had this great doctor, she was already on the mend.

9

twilight sleep

a semiconscious condition induced by the hypodermic administration of morphine and scopolamine. In this state the memory of pain is abolished but not the pain itself.

After her doctor found that she was bleeding internally, they had to do a procedure. They were going to stick something down her throat and into her stomach to see if she had ulcers, which would be good because they can be minor. But if she didn't they would have to go up her and probably that would not be minor.

They said the procedure was pretty routine and usually very safe, but I had worked with sick people before so I asked if there were risks. They said it might tear her but that was very rare. "Were there any other risks?" I asked and they said it could be bad what they found. I was afraid to ask what that might be. I asked what if they didn't do the procedure and they said she would just keep bleeding.

They said she needed to be awake, so they couldn't put her all the way under. They put her under what they called "twilight sleep."

They were going to do it first thing in the morning. She had

13

been in the hospital a couple days to get blood and for "observation." They had been nice about letting me stay with her after visiting hours. I stayed late with her because I didn't want to leave until she was asleep. But as long as I was there she said she couldn't really sleep. She'd close her eyes and sometimes I would too, but in a while she'd think of something she needed to say like where the extra cat food was or where to find the phone number of the man who had started mowing her lawn when she'd become too tired to do so, and one time she said, "Here you are again, taking care of me," because of the times when bad things had happened to her before and I was with her.

We had been acting like there was no need to call anyone else because there was nothing to worry about. We would just call them after it was over and tell them everything was OK.

I remember driving back to her house at night from the hospital. She lived on the other side of the town so I had to drive through the town, which was lit, then out to the country, which was completely dark except for my headlights and the stars.

It was weird to be in her house alone. I had never stayed there without her.

I wanted to get to the hospital early so I could help her get ready, but when I got there she was all ready. A nurse she really liked had helped her into her pre-op nightie and slippers.

She hadn't been able to eat or drink the night before, but she wasn't complaining, she seemed almost excited. She kept saying how much better she already felt because of the blood

14

they had given her. She was acting like the bad part was already over.

They wheeled her into a pre-op room and said it would be a few minutes. Hardly anyone else was around so they let me go in too. She was lying on a gurney. There were a lot of empty ones so I lay down on another one and we giggled like it was nap time and I think we did actually almost sleep. Maybe it was easier to do so during the day, knowing it was light outside, and in a room near one another.

After a while the nurse she really liked came in and when she saw us both on the gurneys she said, "So which one of you is getting this procedure anyway?" and we each pointed to the other and said, "She is," and we all laughed.

My mother was cold so the nurse got her a towel from a cabinet where they were warmed. I could smell it from where I was. It smelled clean and warm and steamy. She wheeled my mother into another room with curtains you can pull around for privacy. After a while we could hear other people coming into other sections and being talked to, then they wheeled my mother in for the procedure and I went out to wait.

I went up to the second floor where people were watching TV. It was a hospital soap opera and I couldn't believe it was on or that anyone was watching it, but there was a guy about thirty staring up at it. A couple of boys who looked like brothers were running around and kicking some toy trucks and making noise. The guy who was watching TV looked like their dad and I wondered about their mother. Maybe she was about thirty too and the way the dad looked, it wasn't like she was having

15

another baby. He wasn't actually watching TV, he was just staring into space.

When the show was over I went back to the waiting room and did nothing for a while.

When her doctor came up to me, he was still in his whites. He was wearing glasses and above them I could see the line where the skin of his forehead had been pressed beneath his surgery cap.

He sat down next to me and said something I forgot when he said the next thing which was that they had found a tumor. He didn't say anything for a few seconds. He was just looking at me to make sure I got it. When I thought about this later, I could tell that he had done this before. He did it kindly, carefully.

He said he couldn't be certain until they got the biopsy back, but "the tumor was probably cancerous."

Then I was doing this thing with the words in my head. I said to myself, He didn't say *she* had cancer, he only said the *tumor* was *probably* cancerous and tumors can be taken out, I thought at exactly the same time. I was making all these fine, picky distinctions in my head. I didn't say anything.

"Do you understand?" he said.

"Yes," I said. I thought I did.

"We can't be certain it's cancerous until we do a biopsy," he said as gently as he could. "But in any event we will need to remove the tumor."

"Yes," I said.

He told me he had told her this while she was still in twilight sleep, then as she was coming out of it, and that they would keep telling her until she was fully conscious and could understand, then I could go in to her. I realized later, too, they didn't want me to tell her because I couldn't have.

She came around more quickly than they thought. When I went in to see her I asked her how she felt and she said OK. I didn't know if I should touch her or if her body still hurt. I stood right next to her and put my hand on the bed.

"They told me what they found," she said.

I wanted to say something. I said, "It's going to be OK."

She did not correct or contradict me. She only said, "I know."

I didn't know what she already knew.

17

metastasis

the spread of disease from one part of the
body to another unrelated to it by conveying
the causal agents or cells through the blood
vessels or lymph channels. This is the mode
by which cancer spreads.

The surgery took less time than

they thought. I had called everyone and my sister and aunt and uncle came down the night before and my mother was happy to see them. My brother wasn't going to be able to get there until after it. My sister and aunt and uncle went out for lunch when the nurses took her in but I couldn't eat. I took a walk around the track at the high school down the road and was back at the hospital in a little bit. I was looking at a magazine, not in a waiting room because it wasn't supposed to go so fast, but then the surgeon, Dr. Kleinman, was there saying, "Hey, I've been looking for you." He was still in his surgery clothes. His hair and forehead were still covered and he had on one of those green shirts that ties in the back. He was holding a folder. I could smell how clean his hands were. He'd just washed them.

"Your mom's in recovery," he said. "She came through the surgery just fine." He smiled, but he sounded tired.

"Thank God," I said, "Thank God."

21

He didn't say anything for a few seconds. He just looked at me. Then he sat down right next to me and opened the folder. There was a line drawing xeroxed on a page. He took a pencil and drew a circle where the tumor had been and a line where he'd cut to remove it. He told me this had gone well. There had been no excessive bleeding and he didn't expect her to have complications in her recovery from the surgery.

Then he didn't say anything because he was waiting for me to be ready to hear the next part.

"What did you find?" I asked.

He made some X marks with his pencil. "We found some abnormal cells here and here . . . and here . . ." He kept making X marks. He made them all over the page. I started to count them then I stopped. He said they'd have to biopsy them to make sure, but it looked like it had spread to all of these places.

"So these are all places where it spread," I said. I pointed to some of the Xs.

"Yes," he said.

I needed to say it out loud. "These Xs are all cancer, right?"

"Yeah," he said, "those are the places we looked."

Which, I realized later, meant *only* the places they had looked, because once they started looking they saw it was everywhere so they didn't have to keep looking.

I made him tell me everything twice and I said it back to him. I needed to say it out loud to get it into me. Then I wrote it down to tell my sister and uncle and aunt.

22

Where it spread was called metastasis. You called them "mets" for short.

After we went over all of it again he asked, "Are you alright?" and he touched my shoulder.

"Yeah," I said.

"I'm sorry," he said. "All we could really do was stop the bleeding."

I could tell he meant it. He had done all he could.

23

incompetence

insufficiency or inability to perform a
function. In legal medicine it refers to an
incapacity or absence of legal fitness, such
as the incompetence of an insane person to
make a valid will.

My mother started making

arrangements as soon as she got out of the hospital. She made an appointment to go to the lawyer and I drove her there. We parked right in front of the lawyer's office and I helped her out of the car and up onto the sidewalk. She had a cane and wasn't used to it.

She signed a will. It started off saying how she was "of sound and disposing mind and memory" and not acting "under duress of any person." She wasn't under duress of another person; she was under duress of being sick. She told the lawyer what to do about her savings and will and retirement. She made a living trust so if she became "incapacitated" or "incompetent"— those were the lawyer's words—all of us kids could write checks and have power of attorney and medical attorney.

A couple months later I was talking to my aunt on the phone. She and her husband were doctors and they had been there for the surgery. When we started talking about them coming to visit again I said they ought to come soon.

My aunt didn't say anything for a second, then she said, she said it sadly, reluctantly, "Have you thought about funeral arrangements?"

When I had packed to come down to my mother's that time, the way I'd been doing for months, I had packed clothes I could wear to a funeral because I was going to stay "for the duration" we called it, that is, until my mother died. My mother had told me she wanted to be cremated.

The hospice people said it was better if you could fill out the paperwork in advance. We filled out what we could, everything except the day and the time of death, which we had to wait for.

It felt terrible to wait for that, as if we wanted it to happen.

I don't remember when I stopped hoping my mother would remain alive. I go over and over this time in my head. I go over and over as if by thinking differently, as if by my remembering what was not I can remake or change what happened. I think "what if—," "what if—," "if only—."

I couldn't see her dying then. I only see her start to die in retrospect. In retrospect she dies over and over again.

I don't remember if there was one day or a certain incident or something someone said or if it was just a gradual slip from actively hoping because I believed, to not allowing myself to think because I was afraid, to realizing that the arrangements we were making were not for her recovery but for final things.

28

tremor

an involuntary quivering or shaking.

Sometimes when I went to see her I
caught a van from the airport. The van took me to a mall then I
waited there for an hour or so until another van got me. It went
via all these other little towns and places that weren't even
towns, just gas stations or rest stops and people would be
waiting for it. I always tried to sit near the back—there were
only a few rows—because I didn't want to talk to anyone.
Sometimes I'd listen to tapes and look out the window. It was
beautiful: wide, clear skies, rich orange and red and blue and
purple sunsets. Rarely cloudy. I could feel hot dry air when the
driver opened the door to let someone in or out. When I got to
my mother's house it was almost night.

I got my bags and paid the driver and walked up the
driveway. The porch light was on and through the slats in the
living room curtain I could see her sitting on the couch. Before,
she would have met me at the airport or come outside and
waved when she heard the van drive up, but she didn't

31

anymore. The front door was ajar. I pushed it open with my bags and said, "Hey Mom!"

She was standing up by then, as if she'd tried to walk to the door to meet me, but couldn't get all the way. She was half leaning, half sitting against the arm of the couch. She was trembling. I dropped my bags and I put my arms around her.

"YOU'RE SHAKING," I said. The way she shook it felt like holding a bird.

"Mom, are you cold? Can I get you something?"

"Oh, no, I'm just fine," she said.

I was wearing a t-shirt. She was wearing a sweater. It was yellow and orange and blue and she looked small in it.

We sat on the couch and she asked me about my trip. I said it was fine, all right. I'd taken it several times by now, but she liked to hear about the other people in the van, about the places we'd dropped them off, or what the sky looked like when we were on the drive.

She'd wanted to stay up to see me in, but she needed to sleep.

I helped her into her nightgown and into bed. By the time I tucked her in she wasn't shaking anymore. I told her to call me if she needed me, then I kneeled down beside the bed and kissed her goodnight.

chemotherapy

the treatment of infection or disease by doses of chemical drugs.

She was supposed to recover from her surgery before she went on chemotherapy. Her doctors said to do it one week a month for six months. My sister was out there for the first round and every night she called me to tell me how it had gone. They went into the oncology clinic at the hospital for most of the day, went home at night, then went back the next day. The first day the only bad thing was it was hard to get the needle in and they had to call someone else to do it. My mother had always had sensitive skin and with her veins getting weak it was hard to get the needle in her. It was huge. But otherwise she was fine. When I talked to her on the phone that night, she said, "I feel fine!" She sounded glad that she'd started it and that it wasn't as bad as she had thought.

The next night when Betty called, she said Mom felt tired and didn't want to talk. Then the next day Mom was feeling nauseous and the next day she was vomiting. The last morning Betty heard her rattling around early in the morning and went

35

in and found Mom trying to rinse out her pillowcase because there was blood all over it. Her mouth was full of sores and she was bleeding from her lips and gums and out of her ears.

WHEN THEY WENT IN for the chemo that day the nurse gave her ice packs and got her some drugs for her mouth sores and told her that happened sometimes but it would go away before the next chemo.

The way the chemo works is to try to kill fast growing cells, like cancer cells, but it also goes after other fast growing cells like you have in your mouth and mucous membranes. Later she bled from her vagina too. The chemo was very strong, which was why you had to not have it for a few weeks between. The worst time was the week after you had it. As it wore off you started to feel not as bad but by the time you felt OK again it was time for your next round. She had three weeks between treatments. She tried to not plan anything for the week of the chemo or for the week or ten days or so after. The time to plan anything was the last week before the next round.

It hurt for her to put anything in her mouth so it was hard to keep her hydrated. Also with the nausea, which never really stopped, even between times, it was hard for her to eat or keep anything down and she was always weak. There was also that huge blue and purple and brown bruise all up and down her arm that took forever to get better. By the time it was just pale green and yellow it was time for the next chemo.

I was there for the next round. The chemo room was one big room with a coffee pot and hot water for tea and cookies on a table and a TV with a VCR. There were big comfy chairs because

36

they had to be there a while. There were other chairs you could drag over to sit next to your person who was getting their IV in the big chair. There were screens you could put between yourself and everyone else but people rarely did. Whenever there were three or four cancer people and whoever came with them, everyone sat around and chatted. They talked about food that worked, like things with ginger, or the flavors of Gatorade or Ensure that they found the least awful. They talked about how good somebody's hair, which could mean either their hair or their wig, looked. The ones who'd been doing this a long time, or once before but now were back, told the new ones about how it was the worst at the start but then you got used to it. They were like a group of old soldiers. Sometimes someone would ask about someone else and one of the nurses might say, "Oh, he moved back to Albuquerque to be with his family," or "Oh, she passed away in August," then you didn't say anything else.

There was an old couple we saw a lot. The woman was getting the chemo, but her husband had had it before and he was always saying how now he was "fit as a fiddle." He was a big guy with a big gut and an L.A. Rams hat. I thought it was amazing, great, that he was fat. My mother had lost a lot of weight. At first she kind of liked this because she used to try to lose weight every now and then, but now her clothes were hanging on her like bags.

The old guy had big red hands that still looked like he worked with them even though he was retired. Sometimes he'd bring wooden toys he had carved or gadgets he would have to explain and leave them there for the chemo room or whoever the nurses wanted to give them to. His wife was still fat and

37

wore a curly wig. When he sat beside her he'd pat her hand and remind her how he was "fit as a fiddle" now.

There was another mother and daughter too. The mom didn't speak any English, only Spanish, so her daughter interpreted for her but she didn't need to much. Two of the oncology nurses were Mexican American and spoke Spanish. Most people spoke a little of it, including Mom and me. I spoke with the daughter in English but not about much. Her mom didn't really look that sick and I didn't want to ask. The nurses were very good about not telling anyone about anyone else's medical details. It was good not to know. I didn't want to hear that someone else only had to come in for three months instead of six or once a week instead of five days or that it hadn't metastasized in them. My mom and the other mom used Spanish, but mostly they just looked at each other and smiled.

My mother and I would sit and watch the people who only came in for one day in the week or only stayed for an hour or so. Most people walked in without any help, but Mom used a cane at first then later she was in a wheelchair.

Around the big chemo room were a couple of other little rooms where you could close the doors so you and your nurse could meet and talk about things with your doctor. The second to the last time we went to one of the little rooms the nurse told the doctor my mother's side effects—her nausea and her bloody mouth and ears and vagina—were bad and she'd become so dehydrated they'd had to bring her in for a night. The doctor decided to give her more time between sessions to recover. So instead of coming back for her next chemo in three weeks, she'd come back in four and they'd see where she was then.

38

Four weeks later when we went back to that little room, the doctor asked her how she was feeling and she told him she still had pain and nausea and that usually when she vomited there was black or bloody stuff in it but that her mouth wasn't bleeding anymore and her hair was coming back.

In the room was the doctor and nurse and Chris and my mother and me. Mom was sitting on the gurney and Chris was sitting behind her. Mom was leaning against Chris like she was the back of a chair. I was leaning against the wall. I was holding this notebook the nurses had suggested we keep. It had when and what my mother ate or drank and if she could keep it down. It had the times and amounts of her meds and how long she slept, like the nurses and doctors said. We were doing everything exactly right, the way they said.

My mother reminded the doctor that she'd been having these side effects to the chemo from the start.

The doctor listened to my mother then was quiet for a while. Then he said that it had been long enough since her last treatment that these things were no longer being caused by the chemo, they were being caused by the cancer.

Later Chris told me that my mother's body had not shifted when the doctor told her this. She said my mother's body was not surprised.

Was my mother relieved to hear out loud what her body already knew?

I think my mother said, "I understand" or "I'm not surprised" or something like that before she was quiet.

I don't remember what anyone else said after that. I think I remember a feeling of something falling.

39

resistance

the natural ability of an organism to
resist microorganisms or toxins produced
in disease.

After the second chemo she was blue and

black from her wrists to her shoulder because her veins were
too weak to hit. It hurt her more than usual when the needle
was going in so they decided to give her a portable catheter. The
porta cath was just a day surgery to put this little thing in her
chest. It was like a hard little bump, a knot beneath her skin. A
few days after she got it, she had to go back for the doctor to
take the dressing off and make sure it had healed.

It was the same doctor who, a couple months before, had
taken out the tumor but told me he couldn't do any more than
stop the bleeding. He was a nice guy with glasses and he seemed
fond of her, like she was like his own mother.

It was a clinic day for him so we went there. Mom was
actually looking forward to it because she hadn't been
anywhere besides the hospital for so long.

She was still walking with a cane. She would have been more

comfortable with a wheelchair but she didn't want one. She wanted to walk on her own two feet, which she could with help.

We parked in a handicapped space. I went around to her side and helped her out of the car and into the clinic.

There was a waiting room with regular sick people. There was an old couple with a guy with his wrist in a bandage, a pregnant woman with a kid, a guy on crutches. There were a couple of mothers with coughing, sniffling kids.

When we came in everyone stared at her. Her face was pale and you could tell that under her hat she was losing her hair. The sick people looked healthy compared to her. They looked fantastic.

I don't know if she knew how she looked. She smiled and some people tried to smile back, but most people looked away. I found my mother a seat and when she sat down I could hear her trying to control her breathing. The few steps into the clinic had taken it out of her. The people next to her leaned away. I went up to the desk and told the receptionist what we were there for and the person sitting next to my mother got up and offered me the seat and I took it. Usually I would have stood but I wanted to sit with her.

After we'd been there awhile people started talking again. People were flipping through magazines and chatting and complaining about the wait. The sniffling, coughing kids started running around.

Because of the chemo, my mother had very low resistance. I went up to the desk and asked the receptionist if I could get a face mask for her. The office was small so you could hear everything. The receptionist was harried. It was near the end of the day but the waiting room was still full and the kids were running around and the receptionist knew I was going to stand over her desk until I got my mother a mask.

My mother had already looked different from how I remembered her. For years her face had been healthy and wrinkled and brown. She'd had a healthy old woman's skin and a healthy old working woman's back. She could haul a fifty-pound bag of compost from the car to the backyard, dig a post hole, bend over and dig around in her squash and tomato plants for hours, lay the bricks on the floor of her greenhouse. Then her face became skinny and sunken and gray from the cancer, then puffy and orange from the chemo. But whenever you would talk to her, she would be animated, smiling or nodding her head because she was eager to fight this thing and she wanted you to see that she was trying to.

The face mask was white and cottony looking, the same thing you'd wear if you were painting or working with fumes. I leaned over her and put it on. I stretched the nylon string wide and lowered it over her cotton cap, her ears and nose and mouth. She adjusted it to fit and when she was finished she looked up at me and said, "Thanks."

It went over almost everything except my mother's eyes. She didn't look like herself anymore. She looked, when it was just her eyes, frightened. She looked in her eyes as if she already knew.

45

baldness

the state of being bald; lacking all or a
significant portion of the natural or usual
covering of hair on the head or sometimes
on other parts of the body.

They said she wouldn't go bald but of course she did.

When she brushed her hair it came out so she started using a comb. She combed it as gently as she could but still it came out, first strands then handfuls then clumps of it like a rabbit or a cat. It was on her pillow and sheets when she woke up in the morning. It was on the towel she used after a bath. It was around the bathtub and in the dryer filter, the back of her chair, the collars of her clothes.

They said it would grow back as soft as a baby's.

She started wearing these winter ski caps she had around. There was a dark green one and a navy one and several others. They were some poly-cotton blend you could buy at Kmart three in a pack like socks. They were cheap and you could throw them in the wash. She'd had them for when she had to run out in the snow for the mail or fill the birdfeeder and also for when we came home because we never had hats and she wanted us not to get cold.

49

Her friend who used to cut her hair gave her a catalogue
where she could order hats. It was a company started by a
cancer survivor who wanted other women to be able to have
nice looking headwear. In the catalogue pictures they looked
like normal women who might have cancer, white and black
middle-aged women. They weren't perfectly shaped girls in
their twenties or models. They looked confident and strong.
They smiled strong, serious smiles. They looked like they had
decided, by gum, to beat this damned thing and that they had.

A few of them actually were bald. Their faces were smooth
and there was that eerie look on their skin when it has no hair,
but they all were smiling. None of them had circles around their
eyes or puffy cheeks from chemo or that yellow-orange look.
None of them had oozy gums or looked like they were about to
vomit blood.

The hats were all natural fabrics, cotton and wool, and
natural dyes and colors. There were dense, heavy weaves for
winter and light, airy ones for summer. The styles had been
inspired by traditional designs that the catalogue described: a
Breton peasant woman's beret, an Elizabethan ladies' cap, an
Australian outback hat with flap, etc., as if you might wear one
even if you weren't bald.

For years my mother and I had gone clothes shopping
together for me: back-to-school outfits when I was a kid, a nice
coat or sweater for Christmas when I was in college. But we
never shopped together for her until she got sick.

We looked at the catalogue and talked about the colors and
styles, which ones looked like her and which ones were

obviously not her. We laughed about some of them. She didn't like the ones with ruffles or ribbons or bows, she liked the simple, classic ones. We talked about what she could wear at home and what she would like to wear when she went out as if she would go out again. We talked about how many to get, how long it would take for her hair to grow back.

She liked one of the berets but only if they had it in light blue, not the peachy color it was in the photo. The cap with the brim would be nice but only in cotton, not wool because that would make her itch. She wondered if they were stretchy and if you could throw them in the wash or had to hand wash or get them dry cleaned.

We ordered several of them. My mother hoped they would arrive before my brother did on his next visit. She said she didn't want to have to wear one of those old ski caps for him and she certainly didn't want him to see her bald.

We have pictures of her at Christmas. She is sitting in a chair stringing cranberries and popcorn for the tree. There's a glass of her Gatorade on the table beside her and she's wearing her dark green Kmart ski cap. The ones we ordered from the catalogue slipped down her smooth shiny head to her browless eyes and didn't keep their shape so she went back to ski caps. When she took them off they were full of flakes and patches of skin. Her skin, despite all the creams and lotions we put on it, was flaking off too.

After she quit the chemo, her hair started coming back. By the time she died, her head was covered with light blonde hair as soft as a baby's.

51

vomit

1. to eject the contents of the stomach.
2. the substance vomited.

She had this pink plastic pan, like a dishwashing pan only smaller, that came from a medical supply store, not a hardware store. It was for vomiting in bed. You or your helper holds it under your head and you vomit into it. It's for when you can't get out of bed because your body isn't strong enough to walk but it is strong enough to spasm and throw up whatever's there.

One of the effects of the chemo was that food smelled horrible to her. There were some smells they told us she wouldn't like— garlic, onions, that kind of thing. There were other things that were supposed to smell good, like ginger, which was supposed to be good for your stomach. Sometimes, though, we'd be cooking something, not garlic or anything we expected to make her feel bad, but she'd shout from her room, "I can smell that!" She didn't want to complain but we knew what she meant. We'd run back to her room and get the pink pan, or she would have it already, and we'd hold it and she'd vomit into it or try to, but

55

only hack and drip saliva because there was nothing in her but her stomach was spasming anyway.

We'd stop cooking whatever it was, open the kitchen door and try to shoo out the smell. After a while we cooked hardly anything and ate in the backyard.

Some kinds of vomit, they said, were like reacting to suggestion, as if somehow she could control it. You were supposed to talk her through it, tell her she didn't really need to vomit and wasn't going to. Sometimes this helped. But that was early on. Later there wasn't anything anyone could do. You'd just hold the bucket and clean her up afterwards.

The vomiting exhausted her. There was no food in her stomach because she hadn't eaten. What was in her stomach was blood, clots and bubbles and strings of it. The black was partially digested. There was phlegm around it sometimes, thick and viscous, white or green. There were thin pink watery strings of it.

I knew each time it happened it was hurting her. It was not only that she was in the process of dying, it was that she was immediately, right then, particularly, acutely, in pain. I saw what happened when her body broke down. Her eyes got wide and frightened looking and the veins on her neck got thick. I wanted to take it from her, but all I could do was hold the bucket under her chin, and hold the back of her head and say, "It'll be over in a second, Mom, it'll be over soon," until it was finished.

It sounded wet and dry at the same time, thick and raspy. Sometimes she was also crying while she did this.

56

After it was over, she would fall back against her pillows and her eyes would close. She would be breathing hard and her face and neck and chest would be covered with sweat. I would wipe with a wet cloth or a baby wipe around her mouth. I would wipe with a sponge inside her mouth then lay a clean moist cloth across her forehead or her cheeks to cool her. Early on we gave her peppermints, those red and white striped discs. We'd unwrap them and hand them to her and she'd suck on them.

Later we had these Q-Tip-like things with little sponges on the ends. You put it in her mouth and she sucked on it then you pulled them out. They came in these little packets, individually wrapped like restaurant straws or toothpicks or lollipops. These were for when the patient could no longer swallow. They were to moisten the mouth.

One of the last things she could do was suck. She sucked it like a baby, open-eyed.

You were supposed to hold it so they couldn't try to swallow it. I remember holding it, the pull of it, the want.

hydrotherapy

the treatment of disease or disability by the external application of water.

My mother used to take long,

hot baths. She'd go in the bathroom with a paperback and
close the door and sit in the tub for what seemed like hours
and read what she called her bathtub books, mysteries by
Agatha Christie, Ngaio Marsh, Dorothy Sayers, Tony Hillerman.
She didn't like the violent ones or the ones with sex. She liked a
good read with quirky characters and colorful settings where
you'd learn something about English village life between the
wars, Aztec history, Flemish food, or Navajo spirituality. She
called this her hydrotherapy.

She always knew the end before it happened.

When she got out of the tub her skin looked pink and soft.
Even if it was early, like seven o'clock, she'd get into her
bathrobe and sit down and watch TV with me or clip and file
her fingernails or read or talk to me.

One time when my sister, who was an art history major, came
home from college I took a picture of her sitting on the toilet,

her head in her hands like Rodin's *Thinker,* and Mom in the
tub beside her, reading a mystery novel. They knew I was
taking the picture and they tried to not laugh. We all thought it
was hysterical. My brother was away at college, too, and I was
still in high school. I was living alone with my mother in a studio
apartment. My mother's hair is long in the picture, dark and
full.

WHEN IT BECAME HARD for my mother to bathe herself
I helped her. At first I sat in the bathroom with her. I sat on the
floor and washed her back and thinning hair and I helped her
get in and out of the tub and I dried her. Her hair was falling
out and her skin was becoming so loose from the weight she was
losing. Along her arms where they had drawn her blood and
put in the chemo were bruises. They were purple and yellow
when they got old, but blue and dark when they were new.

At first I would help her get in and out. She would hold on to
my arm and the side of the tub and lower herself in slowly and I
would help her.

One time I offered to read to her in the tub but she said not
to. Her reading in the tub when we were kids was as much
about getting away from us as it was about reading. Now she
was glad to have us, the children who'd moved away from her,
around her.

"I'm grateful you're here," she said to me. Once she said, "I
feel sorry for people who don't have daughters."

Sometimes we sat and said nothing at all. She sat and soaked
and put in more hot when the temperature cooled and swirled it

in around her. We brought her bubble bath and oils and mineral salts. We got her sea sponges and a blow-up terry cloth pillow to lie back on. When she was finished I'd help her stand and step from the tub and dry her and help put her nightie on.

Later there was the porta cath that you had to be very careful around. You had to keep it dry and clean.

Then later, when she was no longer able to get up if she sat down, we got her a bathseat and installed a moveable shower head.

Finally we washed her with sponges in bed.

We would remove her wet diaper and wipe her with a baby wipe and put on a clean one. We would clean her skin and put lotion on. Some of the time she looked at us but most of the time her eyes were away or closed. Sometimes she would moan and we would think she was trying to say something then this too stopped.

63

hypnophobia

an irrational fear of sleep.

One night she dreamt that she was falling up.

"The ceiling was covered with flowers and I was falling up into them," she said. She said the flowers were white and pretty colored and they smelled clean and sweet but she was afraid. Something was pulling her, lifting her up.

After this dream she was afraid to sleep.

SHE BECAME VERY restless at night. Her doctors gave her drugs for this and I gave them to her with her other meds and talked to her until she was calm then told her goodnight and tucked her in and turned out the light and stayed with her until she slept. I sat by her bed in her father's chair until I heard her breathing evenly. Then I went to the living room to read or to bed in my room across the hall. I kept the light on in the hall the way she'd done for me when I was young. I kept open the door to her room so I could hear her.

Sometimes in her sleep she'd twitch or jolt and cry out loud and I would jump from the couch or stumble from bed and run and try to soothe her. "It's OK, Mom, I'm here, Mom, it's OK." I'd take her hand or smooth her brow and talk to her quietly until she settled down. Sometimes as soon as I touched her she would be calm again.

One night she kept waking up. I'd stay with her until she seemed OK again then I would go back to bed, but then just as I was drifting off, she'd whimper or cry or weep again and I would run across the hall again and touch her arm and tell her it was OK until she settled down.

After this happened several times, I brought the blankets from my bed to her room. I laid them down on the floor beside her bed and whenever she jolted or shouted I reached up to her and touched her arm and said, "It's OK, Mom, it's OK," and she would rest.

I slept on her floor like that for days.

I remember lying in the dark and seeing, in the dim light from the hall, the tops of the medicine bottles lined up along her dresser top and I remembered being sick as a kid and waking up and seeing her there with a glass of water or warm wet wash cloth or whatever it was I needed.

I remember the shape of her body in the bed. Sometimes, when I could only dimly see, she didn't look sick, she only looked, with her even rise and fall of her breath, like someone sleeping. But other times her breath was short and ragged and I could see and hear her hands twitch over the edge of the sheet as if she was looking for something. I would see the shine of

68

sweat on her face as she gurgled and gasped and held her breath. I'd count to ten or twenty and become afraid. Then I would hold my own breath too as if to better hear when she would breathe again then I would be relieved. The nurses said this was Cheyne-Stokes respiration. They said that it began before the end. They said they often died when they were sleeping.

69

morphine

a bitter, white or colorless crystalline alkaloid derived from opium and used in medicine to relieve pain. Principally used in patients dying of inoperable cancer where the problem of addiction does not arise.

When she was at the hospital after her

surgery, they had put her on a morphine drip. They'd cut her open to cut the tumor out then sewed back together the parts of her intestine. The morphine drip hung by the bed in a bag. The liquid looked like anything, a saline solution or glucose.

The morphine was very regulated. The doctor had to order it in advance and a certain guy had to fix the drip and another certain guy had to check it.

She hated being on the drip. The word "morphine" scared her and she hated having that thing always stuck in her arm. Also, she was worried about getting addicted. She asked the doctor if she could and he said there was no danger of that. He didn't say it was because she wouldn't live that long.

One time the drip machine stopped working. The beeper went off and we rang for a nurse but nobody came. The pain was worse. The beeper went off again and we rang again and the beeper kept going off and I ran around the floor trying to get someone. I was saying, "The morphine drip isn't working, my mother is in pain." After a while I found somebody who came and gave her something else, then somebody else came and fixed the machine and the next time it happened they came quickly.

WHEN SHE WENT HOME after the surgery, she was on Roxicet. My brother and I gave it to her. They were big pills she had to swallow. The pain from the surgery was getting better, but she was also getting new pains in weird places like her hip and her shoulder. We wondered if she'd pulled or strained something during the surgery.

She went to a physical therapist who gave her a cane and stretches and exercises and a pillow for her neck but nothing really helped. She was also getting thin and weak and her skin started looking funny.

After a few months we knew the pains were not from the surgery anymore but from the cancer and that the chemo wasn't working.

None of us kids wanted to admit she was ready for hospice care, which you can only go into if you have less than six months to live. The doctors and nurses didn't push us, but then one time when we were talking to one of them and he was talking about "the dying process" we had to stop kidding ourselves. When we talked to her about what the guy had said, she didn't seem surprised. She said she thought it was time.

I think she knew before we did but she didn't want to leave us before she thought we could let her go.

THE DAY AFTER we met with the hospice people they brought a hospital bed and plastic sheets and adult diapers and latex gloves and buckets and sponges and bottles of pills and waste disposal bags and other things you need to die at home.

SHE MOVED FROM Roxicet to Dilaudid, a narcotic they had to call away to El Paso, then Dallas, to get. They sent the ingredients to the pharmacy in Silver City and the pharmacist had to make it up there. The first time this happened was on a weekend and I worried about if he would, but one of the oncology nurses called him and he did it. The nurse told me that she had been the pharmacist's father's nurse when he was dying and the pharmacist would do anything for her.

I got to the pharmacy early and he was still making it up so I had to wait. A clerk was at the cash register and I said, "It's a gorgeous sunset out there." She laughed and said, "You're not from around here, are you?" I said I wasn't and she said it's always the out-of-towners who notice things like the sunset and the air because if you have it every day you just stop noticing it.

A guy came out from the back and handed the bottles to the girl and talked to her and wrote something down. It was the pharmacist. I thanked him for doing this on off-hours and he said, "Sure, no problem." I looked to see if there was anything about him that would tell me his father was dead but I couldn't see anything.

In a couple of days they doubled the Dilaudid, then it kept going up.

It made her nauseous too. She'd vomit whatever she had in

her, which wasn't much. Or she would gasp and heave but there was nothing to come out. Her throat made horrible noises. They put her on anti-nausea pills. One effect of these was constipation so then they put her on stool softeners too. It was like whatever she took, she had to take something else. But it was also that the different parts of her were shutting down. These were stages of "the dying process" we had heard about that time although we never called it that ourselves.

For a while we tried this little machine with pads that gave little jolts of electricity to interrupt the nerves that were sending the pain. You had to put the pads in certain places. The physical therapist came out and adjusted it, but it never really helped so we quit that.

After Dilaudid we went back to morphine but this time pills. The pills were gray and clayey and she picked them up and put them in her mouth and tried to swallow them. Sometimes she was completely aware and alert but other times she'd forget what she was saying or where she was or she'd just stare at us or just stare into space like she was somewhere else or nowhere.

We put the pills in her mouth and waited. Sometimes after a few seconds she would open her mouth to show us that she'd swallowed them and when we didn't see the pills, we'd say, "Good, Mom, you swallowed them!" But then later she'd open her mouth and we could see this gray stuff she hadn't swallowed. It was like the part of her brain that remembered to open her mouth to show us was still working, but not the part of her brain that remembered to swallow.

It looked like clay in her mouth. I put my fingers in and

pulled it out. It felt like dragging a river. I cleaned out her mouth then gave her a clean, wet cloth to suck on.

Then we put her pills into empty capsules and gave them to her like a suppository.

She didn't like to take them that way. We talked about putting her on a drip feed, but she had hated it so much before. Also it would cut into what little mobility she still had. She would have to be more careful about turning over or sitting up in bed or even talking on the phone, which she could still do sometimes.

When she first went on them rectally it hurt her. My sister or one of the nurses would give her meds and then she'd lie on her side for a while to make sure the pills stayed in. I'd go in to read Sherlock Holmes to her to get her mind off it. She joked about this, called it her Holmes Distraction Therapy. I'd read until she asked me to stop or until she slept. Sometimes I read long after she slept, as if she could still know I was there.

Other times she seemed completely unaware and you just put them in and turned her back over.

Later they also put her on fentanyl patches, which were like nicotine patches except for pain. We put them on her like Band-Aids and they released drugs into her and we took them off seventy-two hours later. Her doctor started her with twenty-five milligrams but that went up and there were patches all over her. When you took them off, no matter how careful you were, her skin was red. Her skin was tender anyway, and you knew it hurt to take them off even if she didn't indicate she was aware. You tried not to put the new ones down where the old ones had been but after a while they had been all over her. They looked like grafts.

After she got where she was out of it all the time and wouldn't be aware of it, we discussed putting her on a drip feed but by then the nurses said it would only be a few days. Also, I think we all needed some activity we could do, like counting and divvying the pills into their capsules and putting them in her, as if something we could do would help.

hallucination

a visual delusion such as seeing relatives who
are long dead, reptiles, spiders, or crawling
monsters that are not actually present.

One night when I had gone back home

for a few days, my sister called me on the cordless phone from Mom's backyard. We were doing this more because we never knew when she would wake up and hear us and we were saying things we didn't want her to hear. Sometimes it seemed her hearing had gotten more acute. She'd hear things we didn't think she could. Sometimes she heard things the rest of us couldn't.

My sister had bought the cordless phone a few months earlier because if Mom heard the phone ring, she wouldn't just let it ring or take a message, she'd try to run for it. In any event, she didn't get to use the cordless much.

It was late when my sister called and she was keeping her voice down low. I could picture her out back, under the dark New Mexico sky, the huge white stars far above her. I wondered if she had the cigarettes. Neither of us really smoked anymore but one night when Mom was back in the hospital, we'd driven home via the drive-thru liquor store, which we totally loved the idea of because it was so horrible, and got a six-pack of Corona and some cigarettes, something really shitty like Merit Lights, and taken them home to Mom's and gone out back and smoked and drank and were bad girls together. There was something about smoking together—while our mother, who had smoked a couple packs a day until her late fifties and was lying tonight in a hospital bed across town dying of cancer—that was like standing up to it, like giving the finger and saying "fuck you" to the cancer. It was a stupid thing to do, but it let us get loud and laugh and feel better for a while. So my sister was calling me from where we'd gotten loud and she sounded scared.

She told me she had put Mom to bed then gone to bed herself but before she was asleep Mom called her and she went into Mom's room and Mom said, slightly perturbed, but matter-of-fact, "Will you please take that monkey out of my room?"

The monkey chattering on her night table was keeping her awake.

I don't know if my sister tried to tell our mother that there was no monkey, or if my sister acted like she saw it, if she picked it up or coaxed it away with a peanut or a toy, or if she trapped it or chased it or whatever you'd do with a monkey, but after a while the monkey left and my mother said now she was finally going to be able to get some sleep.

Our mother was on a ton of drugs, more and more of them as things went on: pain meds, narcotics, dope. But seeing the monkey was more than the drugs. It made us understand that her brain was shutting down. What our mother needed to know of our world was less and less. The world she needed to know of was another. It was a world we could not understand or go to. She was going there without us.

That is, I hoped that what my mother was seeing was a place that she could go to that was good. I didn't want for her to simply end. I wanted her to be relieved of what her life here had become by going somewhere there was solace, mercy, rest.

We tried to figure out why it was a monkey. Our mother hated monkeys. When I was a kid and we went to the zoo, which wasn't often, Mom never went into the primate house. She didn't like any of them, gorillas or apes, or chimpanzees with their red naked butts, but mostly, because they were so human, the monkeys. She thought they looked dirty, always picking at their lice and skin. She hated how they looked so almost human, like deformed little hairy men. I think it all went back to *The Wizard of Oz*.

That was her favorite movie. She'd read the books when she was a kid and still had early editions of them, including the really obscure ones like *Tik-Tok of Oz*, *Ozma of Oz* and other ones I don't remember the names of, but it was the movie that really got her. She was ten years old when it came out. It was the beginning of color in the movies and she told me how when it went from the black and white of Kansas to the color of Oz it was completely, absolutely magical. She had never—no one had ever—seen anything like it before and it was wonderful.

She didn't live in Kansas, but in a place enough like it. Oklahoma was flat and dry and had tornadoes and big, kind, simple men who worked as farmhands and my mother had a

83

great imagination. My aunts tell stories of my mother as a little girl listening to the radio, acting out all the parts and doing all the voices. They tell about stories my mother made up and plays my mother performed. It's like she was able to get right inside whatever she heard on the radio, or whatever book she was reading. No one was surprised when she went away to college and majored in speech and drama and radio. But even after she was older, when she was a mother to three full-grown kids, and the monkey scenes in *The Wizard of Oz* came on the TV, she had to leave the room.

My sister and I wondered if this was why it was a monkey. But even in this we were pretending. We were still hoping that however much she was diminishing, our mother was still the way we used to know.

SHE BEGAN TO SPEAK to people who were not there.

Once her voice went high like a child's voice. Though she was old and bald and her skin hung loose and her cheeks sunk over her toothless mouth, she suddenly sat up and said, in a singsong voice like a girl playing hide and seek, "Where are you?"

Then with sudden strength she pushed herself up from her pillows, threw the covers back and swung out her pale, skinny legs from the bed and shot to the floor. I didn't stop her. I followed her.

"Where are you?" She looked around the bed. "Where are you?"

"I'm here," I said, "beside you."

She kept moving as if she hadn't heard me. She dashed to the

84

corner with more energy than she'd had for weeks and looked behind the bookshelf. "Are you here?"

"I'm beside you," I said.

She laughed, "Not *you!*" then went on breezily, "I know where *you* are."

Then she said again in that child's voice, "Where are you? Where are you?"

I followed her as she scurried around her room.

"Are you there?" She looked behind the door. "Are you there?"

Her nightgown was loose around her. Every day she was losing more weight.

She opened and closed the door. "Are you there? Are you there? Where are you?"

My mother was back in her childhood.

I tried to imagine her there, a girl in the 1930s playing hide and seek with her sisters.

LATER, WHEN SHE could not get out of bed, she asked me once, "Who are all these people who are coming to help me?"

"Jo Marie?" I said, naming one of her hospice nurses.

"No." She sounded puzzled.

"Michael?" Another nurse.

"No." Her brow was furrowed. Her hairless skin looked soft.

"Who are all these people who are coming to help me?"

I named the rest of her nurses, then her doctors and sisters and neighbors.

None of them were who she meant.

85

After a while she got quiet and we just sat there.

She was staring intently, seeing something.

"It's Daddy," she said. "It's Daddy and other people I don't know. They're coming to help me."

My mother's father, whom she had always loved, had died nearly thirty years before. A few weeks earlier, when my mother still had periods of lucidity, my brother had sat beside her bed and she had told him she'd been dreaming of her father. She dreamt her father was standing near, in front of her. He didn't say anything, just smiled. She said she thought he was waiting for her.

I want to think that how her dying looked to us, the trembling and sweating of her body, was only the body's trial, but that some other part of her was helped by something else. I want to believe that my mother was helped by something kind. Perhaps it was her father who came to help.

86

illusion

a perception that misinterprets the object
perceived; a false perception.

One morning she awoke with a

start. She sat straight up in bed and said, "Is everything ready?"

My brother and I were with her. We'd been watching her
sleep. Her skin was shiny, her eyes were bright, her hands were
scrabbling across the sheet.

"Is everything ready?" she asked again. Her voice was
livelier than it had been for days, impatient as a child. "Is
everything ready?"

"Yeah," my brother said. "Everything's ready, Mom."

"Oh good." She sounded relieved. When she lay back against
the pillows she looked old again. She didn't have her dentures
in. I fluffed the pillows around her. "Good . . ." she kept
saying, "good . . ." Then she drifted off, then just stared.

Her eyes were cloudy and her hands were limp on the sheet,
then suddenly she sat up again and was doing that scrabbling
thing with her hands. "Is everything ready? Is everything
ready?" She sounded frantic.

89

I looked at my brother then back at her. She kept talking in
short, quick sentences.

"Everything's ready, Mom. Everything's taken care of," my
brother said.

I straightened her cap and wiped her face clean with a baby
wipe. I put my hand on her forearm and her twitching slowed.
"Yeah, Mom. Everything's all taken care of. You don't have to
worry about anything."

She looked relieved for a second but then she just got that
blank look again.

My brother went on casually. "Yeah, Mom, Becky's all ready,
all taken care of." My mother had started calling me this, my
childhood name, again. "Aren't you, Bec?"

"Yeah, I am. I'm doing totally fine. Everything's great with
me. You don't have to worry about me, Mom."

"Betty's great too, Mom," my brother said cheerily.

"She really is," I added. "She's doing really great. Totally
great. Great job, great kid, great friends. She's just doing
great, Mom."

My brother said, "I'm doing great too, Mom. We all are. We
are all doing great. Everything's great with all of us."

I couldn't tell how much she heard or understood.

"Ready to go?" she asked.

"Ready when you are," he said. He sounded like she used to
sound when we were young and eager to be going to a movie or a
park or a baseball game of my brother's or on a road trip. She
used to make our road trips, when she would drive us across
the country to follow our father's work, into games. We'd play
the License Plate Game or Road Signs or Scenery. I didn't

90

know for years how hard these trips had been for her. I didn't know how liberated, how happy, she later felt when she was able to go on driving trips to places she wanted to see, not just to follow our father.

"Yep," my brother said cheerily, the way she would have once. "Everything's ready to go."

"When." She said it more like a statement than a question.

"Whenever you want, Mom!" Now I was sounding cheery too, the way you do with a baby to make them feel safe even though they don't understand what you're saying.

"Yeah, Mom. Whenever you want is fine by us," my brother said.

". . . How about Saturday?" she said.

"Saturday? You wanna go Saturday, Mom?"

She looked at us. Her eyes were wide.

"Saturday OK with you, Bec?"

"You bet," I said. "Everything's taken care of. Bill's got all the money stuff worked out and Momma Kitty is coming with me and Chris—"

"Who?" These names of her cat and my partner, names from more recently in her life, were puzzling to her.

"Everything's OK," my brother jumped in. "We're all ready whenever you are."

"Are we all packed?"

"You're packed, Mom, but all of us aren't going, just you. But you've got everything you need."

"Oh, thank you. . . . Well, how about Saturday? There won't be so much traffic on Saturday . . ."

"Whenever you want, Mom. Saturday would be fine."

This took place on a Wednesday or a Thursday, I can't remember exactly, but at least a couple of days before Saturday. Everyone thought she would be dead by then. My brother and I were acting as if, were hoping, when she talked to us like this, that on some level our mother understood that, for us, it was OK for her to leave. She had always worried, especially after our father left, about us feeling abandoned. She worried about money, about how to support us. She didn't want us to feel alone or left. We hoped, we wanted to believe, that we could let her know she didn't need to worry about us anymore, that she could leave. We wanted to believe she could, somehow, decide or have some choice about the time, that her dying could be good, in her right time. We wanted to believe there was some thing that she could know and that she was trying to tell us.

She didn't die that Saturday. She lived days longer than anybody thought. Then when she died it was not peacefully or easy, it was hard. As long as she tried to put it off, and though we had told her we were ready, we were not.

unction

the act of anointing, as in medical treatment
or a religious ceremony.

A few days before my mother died, I

said to my sister, "I want to prepare the body with you."

We were in my mother's living room. Our mother was in her bedroom down the hall where she was dying. She was asleep or resting or whatever it was, on morphine and Haldol and other drugs the names of which I no longer remember. None of the drugs were to cure anymore. They were only to comfort.

She lay in the bed in her room down the hall while my sister and I sat whispering in her living room. It was late at night and though our mother was asleep and couldn't hear us, we acted as if she could, as if we might wake her. We might have once. She was always a very light sleeper, especially around her children: she was vigilant. So my sister and I were acting as we'd been raised, to whisper when we were near to somebody sleeping.

We'd begun to whisper a lot in my mother's house. Before we knew how sick she was when we talked to her docs on the phone, sometimes we'd whisper. "She picks at her food," we'd say. "Should I make her eat?" "The pain is still in her shoulder. Should I give her another pill?"

When our relatives called early on, we'd whisper little triumphs. "She ate four bites of mashed potatoes today." "She only vomited twice!" Or "We walked her out to her garden today."

Later, when she was sick unto death, we'd whisper to them, "If you want to come see her, come soon."

THE NIGHT MY MOTHER died, my sister came into our room and said, "Chris?" and I shot out of bed. I went to my mother's room and touched her, her face and her pulse, and I saw her face and I said to my sister and Chris, "She's dead." Chris touched my mother and said she was. She was dead.

I don't remember what I did. Did I cry out loud or say something? Did I lean over my mother and kiss her? I don't remember. I remember my sister getting onto the bed and holding my mother and crying and saying "Momma." When she got up, Chris lay beside my mother too and held her and thanked my mother out loud for loving her. I remember my sister, either with something she said or a gesture, asking did I want to lie with my mother and hold her good-bye, but I couldn't.

Her face was yellow and waxy and smooth. Her cheeks were flat and her eyes were sunk and one of them was open. I tried to close it. Her head was shiny and almost bald, but with a little fuzz of hair where it had started to grow back when she stopped the chemo. It looked like a baby's, soft and white.

FOR DAYS MY SISTER and I and Chris, after she arrived, had gathered things for my mother—rose petals from a bouquet from the boys, sage and basil and rosemary for remembrance from her garden. Betty had brought some mugwort from an herbalist in town who told her it would bring clear dreams to the dead. We'd found an old green glass pitcher with a cork in the top and an old bronze vase of my grandfather's.

My mother's body was covered with sweat. We'd been changing her sheets and the night shirt she was wearing several times a day, but she'd break into sweats as we changed them. Sweat would pour down her body. I didn't know how she could have so much when she hadn't been able to drink at all for days.

We washed my mother with warm, clean, sweet-smelling water. I remember the bowl with the water in it, and my sister and Chris and I each dipping our hands, or our hands and a cloth, into the bowl, then washing my mother's skin. We took turns holding the bowl and took turns washing.

Her body was hairless as a girl and it was smaller. She'd lost so much weight and her skin was loose. But when we washed her, lifting her hand, her arm, her foot, her neck, she gave to us. The tension in her body, how it was stiff and clenched and could not bend or be turned easily the last days of her life, the twitching and the rigidness her body had had for days, had been released.

97

The doctors and the hospice workers had said she was past feeling, that the twitches and groans that came from her were involuntary. Her brain stem was only functioning at the very lowest level, to make her lungs breathe and her blood circulate. They told us she was not aware and that her body could not feel anything.

But it was hard to see her twitch, and hear her throat and mouth make noises that sounded almost human, almost like speech, as if she was trying to tell or ask or beg us for something, for mercy perhaps.

We washed our mother's body and we talked to her. Her body was limp and gave to us and we washed her slowly and tenderly, as if she could still feel us, or feel us again. We washed her skin and told her that we loved her and we'd remember her. We thanked her for her life, for being good to us and kind. We told her that her body's pain was over. We told her we'd take care of things. She'd worried about things when she was alive, that she had left a burner on or hadn't locked a door. She worried about her children, if we'd eaten enough or were warm and safe, if we felt cared about and loved. We told her everything was fine, that things were taken care of, that she could rest.

Her skin looked flat and yellowish and felt beneath my hands like wax, still warm and soft and pliable.

We turned her over and changed the sheets then covered her with jasmine-scented oil. It was massage oil I had brought to her one time. My mother had never had a massage before she got sick and didn't really want one at first, but she got used to them. Every night whoever was with her, my sister or brother or me, would rub her shoulders and back and neck, her legs and arms and feet to help her sleep.

I poured the oil in my sister's hands, then Chris poured it into mine and hers and we covered my mother's body with oil. The room began to smell so clean. Our hands were soft and slippery. I remember the touch of my mother's skin, beneath my fingers and hands, the way she felt.

We poured red wine into a cup and drank. Then my sister put her hand in the cup and touched her fingers to our mother's mouth and spread the wine along her lips.

We covered her with flower petals and herbs we got from her garden. We tucked the charms her son and her grandson had made into her hands. We wrapped the clean white sheet and then her father's woolen blanket around her. We covered the flesh that had carried her, the body she had borne, that she had birthed us from, the body from which we had washed the final sweat. When this was done we lay her down in her bed alone as if she could rest until morning.

99

cremation

the burning of dead bodies.

The next morning we called the funeral

parlor and a guy came out. He was young, a big husky Mexican American guy dressed in a nice suit and shiny black shoes. He smelled fresh and clean, like aftershave. We had just gotten out of our pajamas or the shower. We were wearing jeans and shirts and my sister's hair was still wet. We'd slept, probably the best we'd slept in ages, but there was something not quite awake about us, like we were all in a daze. It wasn't until after the funeral guy left that I saw I was wearing my slippers.

The guy was gentle and soft-spoken and let us take our time. My sister's face was puffy and red from crying. Chris was calm and I was practical, like "We need to do this." "I think we ought to do this." Jo Marie, the hospice nurse, was there too. We'd called her earlier, about eight or something. I remember Chris and my sister and I discussing if we'd wake Jo Marie up but she'd told us to call her any time and given us her home phone. She was expecting it.

My mother had died in the middle of the night and we'd prepared the body. We'd wrapped her in a sheet and then in her father's favorite blanket as if to comfort her. We left her face uncovered as if she could breathe. Her face was beautiful. It looked like her exactly but also not, a way I wonder if I always could have seen but didn't. Her face looked calm and light and full of ease and rest.

We'd done all this by candlelight and when we were done we blew out the candles and opened the window. When she was sick we had been careful to never let the room get cold. But after she was dead we could open the window and let in the air the way she used to love. My sister remembered an old saying about you open the window to let out the spirit of the dead.

After we did this, as if we could rest, my sister went to bed and Chris and I stayed up and watched a video of Sherlock Holmes my mother had taped. My mother loved that show. She'd taped almost all of them. I drank the rest of the wine and ate the rest of this cake a neighbor of my mother's had made and brought over. It was like bread with fruit in it, very hearty and sweet. It was some special kind of bread that meant something but I couldn't remember what. I ate the bread and drank the wine and watched TV then went to bed with Chris. I didn't think I would sleep but I did. We all did. Everyone could rest.

So when the funeral guy got there in the morning the body was prepared so all we had to do was take her out.

You were supposed to put the body on this stretcher and wheel it out of the house. The funeral guy was looking at the

104

hall and trying to figure out the best way to get the stretcher in and the body out and I said, "Can we carry her? I think we should carry her out." I tucked the sheet and blanket around my mother's face to cover her. My sister and Chris and me and my mom's next door neighbor, her best friend, got on either side of the bed and put our hands underneath her to carry her. I could feel the wool of her father's blanket. He'd had it when he was a young man in the first world war. We lifted her out of the bed.

She was cold by then. I could feel that through the blanket. She didn't feel like a person. She was stiff. This made her easier to carry in one way though she was heavier than I thought.

We carried her out of her room and down the hall, through her living room and out of the house.

Outside the day was beautiful. It was bright and clear and the air was crisp. It was early Sunday morning.

We carried her to the driveway where the van was backed up. The guy opened the back of the van and we put her in on this cot thing. The guy strapped her to it and locked the wheels on the bottom. The wheels were so you could roll them out easily to where they'd burn.

When we put her in, the blanket slipped and you could see the top of her head. There was just a little bit of hair and it was pale. It looked like a baby's head, like a baby pushing out of its mother getting born. I went up and tucked the blanket back together over the head as if to keep it from getting cold.

After a while somebody thanked the guy and he closed the back of the van and we couldn't see her anymore.

105

remains

1. a dead body. 2. what is left.

It takes most of a day. You have to make an

appointment because they can only do so many at a time. And in our case, the undertaker had to drive the body to another town because there was not a crematorium in her town. I think the undertaker and the people who owned the crematorium were cousins. Each person we spoke to about any of this was patient and kind. We knew our mother would have liked them, decent people running honest family businesses.

I wanted to go with her. I said I'd drive along behind the van to the crematorium. I wanted to wait with her the way I had waited for her at the surgery and then at the doctor's appointments and then the times when she was trying to sleep or to keep something down or for some pain to pass, some drug to kick in that sometimes did but sometimes didn't. I wanted to wait with her while her body burned.

The undertaker didn't say I couldn't. He only said there wasn't a waiting room or anything like that set up. No one said

109

anything for a while, then I realized that I could not wait with her anymore.

We watched the van drive off and went back in the house. The nurse had made the bed and it looked nice. It didn't look like someone dead had just been taken from it.

After a while I said, "Let's go up to the Ruins." They were these old cliff dwellings my mother had loved. We hadn't brought any of our hiking stuff down with us so we put on sweaters and coats and scarves and gloves of my mother's. We packed some picnic stuff and drove a couple of hours into the mountains. We drove her car.

There was snow on the side of the roads and some places on the road where the sun hadn't reached. The sky was clear and blue and the air was cold. I wore my mother's driving gloves as I drove. I put on her winter jacket when I got there.

I'd been there lots before with her. It was one of her favorite places.

When Chris and I got there in the afternoon we didn't see anyone else around. We bundled up and started up the trail. There was snow on it. It didn't seem like too much but we couldn't know if there was a lot at the top.

We weren't very far in when we saw a National Park person coming down the trail toward us.

"There's lots of snow up ahead," she said.

"Don't tell me we can't use the trail today." I sounded frantic.

"No, you can hike today. Just be careful."

She sounded calm, especially after I'd been so bristly. She looked at me like, Are you OK?

110

I said, "My mother died last night and this was one of her favorite places so we had to come here." I said it quickly.

She looked at me for a second then said, "Oh God. I'm so sorry."

"We really want to go up there today." I nodded up at the Ruins. I wanted to say something else but I didn't know what. The park woman looked at Chris then at me again and we turned up the trail.

We hiked for a long time before we got to the ladder. We climbed it, our hands and feet on the smooth, flesh-polished wood. At the top, where we could go into the rooms, we were above the trees. Nothing was blocking the sun from us there. It fell right on us, bright and clear. We took off our scarves and jackets and gloves and we were warm.

The Gila Cliff Dwellings, about forty rooms, were built by descendents of the Mogollon around 1200. These people grew corn and beans and hunted and gathered wild plants. They made nets and snares and baskets and wooden tools and pottery. There were maybe ten to fifteen families living at the cliff dwellings at any one time. In the early 1300s they left. No one knows where they went or why. The year before she got sick, my mother had done volunteer work with an archeology crew at a different Mogollon site. She learned, she told me, that the only remains these people left were some tools, some pieces of broken pottery and these ruins.

THE NEXT DAY WE went to pick up the remains.

They were in a box. The box was plastic, almost a cube but not quite, brown and sturdy. It had her name on it and a date.

111

I can't remember and I don't want to look to see if it was the date of her death or of the day that her body was burned.

Inside the box was a plastic bag, thick, like a freezer bag. In the bag were the ashes. The ashes were mostly gray and black and white but not all of them. Among them there were flecks of blue, like the egg of a bird, or green like an after-dinner mint, and brownish gold like sand. Some of the ashes were pretty and I wondered what they were.

They were also not of uniform size, though all of them were small. There was nothing in there to recognize.

We put our hands in the bag and touched the ashes. The texture of them was various. From smooth and almost papery, to grainy or gritty like sand, to powdery like a butterfly's wing. The ash stuck to and colored our hands. I remember streaks of it on my hands, the pads of my fingers blackening, how it gathered and caked in lines of my palms. They were not like the ashes from a fireplace, soft and uniform or with charcoal pieces or pieces of half-burnt wood. The ashes were dry. They were neither warm nor cold.

A friend of hers had given to her a homemade ceramic pot with a lid. On the side was a design of a bird. We put the ashes in it and took it to another favorite place of hers. She'd taken us there for picnics and to gather wildflowers to dry and smooth, round, waterworn stones for her backyard pond. It was a canyon carved deep in the mountains by a spring.

We walked out to the end of it and ate the picnic lunch we'd packed and we thought and talked about her. After we'd finished eating and been quiet for a while we all dipped our

112

hands into the pot and pulled out a handful of ashes and scattered them into the canyon below us. Then after a while my brother, whom she had watched and cheered at baseball games for years when he was a kid, picked up the pot, as all of us had asked him to do, and threw it far across to the other side of the canyon. We heard it crack, then saw the puff of the last of the ashes released. They floated, suspended, until they sank. We watched the air in front of us go smoky and gray to clear, then we looked down below us. We looked down past the struggling brush, then deeper, past the lichen-covered stones. We looked to where the earth had cracked, a place we could not see.

There the water carried her away.

113